GLUTATHIONE FOR BEGINNERS

Unlocking Health And Vitality, The Comprehensive Guide To Boost Your Immunity, Detoxify Your Body, Combat Aging, And Rejuvenate Your Cells

Georgette Lockett

DISCLAIMER

The author of this book is not affiliated, associated, endorsed, sponsored, or approved by any company or individual. The views and opinions expressed in this book are solely those of the author and do not necessarily reflect the official policy or position of any entity.

The author hereby disclaims any relationship, collaboration, or partnership with any company or individual mentioned in this book. Any references to products, services, or individuals are provided for informational purposes only and should not be construed as an endorsement or recommendation.

Readers are advised to exercise their own judgment and discretion when applying the information provided in this book. The author shall not be held responsible for any actions taken by readers based on the content of this book.

This book is intended for general informational purposes only, and the author makes no representations or warranties of any kind, express or implied, about the completeness, accuracy, reliability, suitability, or availability of the information contained herein. Any reliance on the information in this book is at the reader's own risk.

The author reserves the right to update, change, or modify any information in this book without notice. It is the responsibility of the reader to verify any information before taking any actions based on the content of this book.

By reading this book, the reader acknowledges and agrees to the terms of this disclaimer.

Table of Contents

INTRODUCTION

Glutathione is an amino acid tripeptide composed of three amino acids: cysteine, glutamic acid, and glycine. It is an important antioxidant that is created naturally in the body and plays an important function in cellular defense against oxidative stress. When there is an imbalance between the generation of free radicals and the body's capacity to neutralize them, oxidative stress arises. Glutathione is a potent antioxidant that scavenges free radicals and protects cells from harm.

Importance In Human Health

The importance of glutathione in human health cannot be emphasized. Glutathione is engaged in a variety of vital actions inside the body apart from its involvement in countering oxidative stress. It helps the immune system, assists in detoxification processes, and is necessary for red blood cell integrity. Furthermore, glutathione is important in the control of many cellular activities, including DNA synthesis and repair.

Purpose And Scope Of The Guide

The purpose and scope of this guide are to give a full overview of glutathione, including its structure, functions, sources, and influence on health. It will investigate the methods by which glutathione functions as an antioxidant, as well as its involvement in cellular health. The guide will also go into glutathione sources, both dietary and inside the body, as well as variables that might alter its levels.

Furthermore, the book will look at the possible advantages of glutathione supplementation and how it might help with general well-being. Along with the benefits, it will discuss the hazards, contraindications, and precautions connected with glutathione usage.

Readers can anticipate a thorough investigation of glutathione, from its chemical structure to its influence on human health, which will provide vital insights for anyone interested in maximizing their health and understanding the function of antioxidants in the body.

CHAPTER 1

Understanding Glutathione

Definition And Structure

Glutathione is a tripeptide composed of the amino acids glutamine, cysteine, and glycine. Its chemical structure enables it to function as an antioxidant inside the body. This chemical is created spontaneously in human cells and plays an important function in a variety of physiological processes.

Glutathione, also known as GSH, is a strong antioxidant found in the majority of the body's cells, tissues, and organs. Its chemical structure is distinguished by a distinct tripeptide arrangement. The sulfhydryl (thiol) group in its cysteine residue is critical to its antioxidant capabilities. Because of its ability to give electrons, it is excellent in neutralizing dangerous free radicals and reactive oxygen species (ROS).

Function In The Body

Its principal role in the body is to protect cells from oxidative damage. Glutathione serves as the first line of defense against free radicals, which are unstable chemicals that cause cellular damage. It helps prevent cellular damage, protects the integrity of cellular components, and promotes general cell health by neutralizing free radicals. It also aids in the elimination of toxins, heavy metals, and toxic chemicals during detoxification processes inside the liver.

Antioxidant Properties

Glutathione's antioxidant qualities are critical for cellular health. It scavenges free radicals, protecting lipids, proteins, and DNA from oxidative damage. This safeguard is critical in lowering the risk of a variety of illnesses, including cardiovascular disease, neurological disorders, and some malignancies. Furthermore, it aids in the regeneration of other antioxidants such as vitamins C and E, therefore strengthening the body's antioxidant defense system.

Understanding the function of glutathione in cellular defense and its antioxidant capacities gives a solid basis for appreciating its significance in general health and well-being.

CHAPTER 2

Biosynthesis Of Glutathione

Enzymatic Pathways

Glutathione (GSH) is a tripeptide made up of three amino acids: glutamine, cysteine, and glycine. Its production takes place intracellularly, largely in the cytoplasm of cells, via a strictly controlled enzymatic mechanism. Two ATP-dependent enzymatic stages are involved in the synthesis.

1.-GCS (Gamma-Glutamylcysteine Synthetase):

• This enzyme catalyzes the first and most important step in the production of glutathione. It forms -glutamylcysteine by combining glutamate and cysteine.

• This stage is highly controlled and critical in determining glutathione synthesis rate.

2. Synthetase of Glutathione:

• Following the production of -glutamylcysteine, the enzyme glutathione synthetase attaches glycine to the -glutamylcysteine molecule, completing glutathione synthesis.

Factors Influencing Synthesis

Several variables may alter glutathione production in the body:

• **Nutritional Availability:** Substrate availability, such as cysteine, the rate-limiting precursor for glutathione synthesis, has a substantial influence on glutathione production. Because of its availability in the diet, cysteine is often the limiting factor.

• **Enzyme Activity:** The rate of glutathione production is determined by the activity and expression of the enzymes involved in the synthesis process, notably -glutamylcysteine synthetase.

• **Oxidative Stress:** Increased oxidative stress might increase glutathione demand, possibly altering its manufacture to combat oxidative damage.

• **Genetic Factors:** Variations in the genes encoding glutathione synthesis enzymes may impair an individual's ability to effectively manufacture glutathione.

Dietary Sources

Although glutathione is poorly absorbed when consumed orally, several dietary components help to produce it:

• **Foods rich in Cysteine:** Foods rich in cysteine or its precursor amino acids, such as cysteine and methionine, may help glutathione production indirectly. Poultry, eggs, dairy, legumes, and some grains are examples.

• **Vitamins and minerals:** Micronutrients such as vitamin C, vitamin E, selenium, and folate indirectly enhance glutathione production by assisting in the recycling of oxidized glutathione back to its active state and by increasing the activity of enzymes involved in glutathione synthesis.

Understanding the enzymatic routes, variables affecting synthesis, and dietary sources sheds light on the complicated processes behind glutathione formation in the body, emphasizing its relevance in cellular health and redox equilibrium.

CHAPTER 3

Health Benefits Of Glutathione

Cellular Protection

Glutathione is the body's main antioxidant. Its major role is to neutralize free radicals, preventing oxidative stress in cells. Free radicals, which are created during metabolic processes or as a result of external causes such as pollution or UV radiation, may damage cells and DNA, resulting in a variety of illnesses and aging. Glutathione scavenges free radicals, avoiding cellular damage and promoting cell health overall.

Detoxification

Detoxification is another important function of glutathione. It binds to hazardous compounds such as heavy metals, contaminants, and some medications, converting them to a form that the body can readily discard. Glutathione works inside the liver, a vital detoxification organ, aiding in the breakdown and elimination of pollutants.

Immune System Support

Glutathione is essential for keeping a healthy immune system. It improves the activity of immune cells including lymphocytes and natural killer cells, which helps the body fight infections and disorders. Low glutathione levels may impair the immune system, leaving the body more vulnerable to sickness.

Anti-Aging Properties

As an antioxidant, glutathione aids in the fight against oxidative stress, a major cause of aging. It may reduce the aging process by lowering oxidative damage to cells and tissues, encouraging healthier skin, greater organ function, and overall vitality.

Glutathione research continues to increase, revealing its promise in a variety of medicinal sectors. However, although supplementary glutathione may seem to be a straightforward remedy, its oral absorption might be restricted. Ongoing research is looking at ways to boost glutathione levels via lifestyle changes, dietary choices, and tailored supplementation.

CHAPTER 4

Glutathione And Disease Prevention

Role In Chronic Diseases

Glutathione is essential in the prevention and treatment of a variety of chronic disorders. Its antioxidant qualities are critical in neutralizing free radicals and lowering oxidative stress, which has been linked to the development of a variety of ailments such as cardiovascular disease, neurological disorders, cancer, and diabetes.

• **Cardiovascular Diseases:** Oxidative stress has a crucial role in heart disease. Glutathione protects cardiac tissues and blood arteries from oxidative damage, possibly lowering the incidence of heart attacks, strokes, and atherosclerosis.

• **Neurodegenerative Disorders:** Oxidative stress and the buildup of damaged proteins have been related to diseases such as Alzheimer's, Parkinson's, and Huntington's. The capacity of glutathione to combat oxidative damage may provide neuroprotective benefits, perhaps reducing the advancement of certain disorders.

• **Cancer Prevention:** Glutathione aids in the detoxification of toxins as well as the immune system's monitoring of malignant cells. According to some studies, keeping appropriate glutathione levels may reduce the incidence of some malignancies.

• **Diabetes and Metabolic Disorders:** Insulin resistance and diabetes complications are exacerbated by oxidative stress. The function of glutathione in reducing oxidative stress may aid in the management of diabetes and its consequences.

Potential Therapeutic Applications

Because of its many activities, there is rising interest in using glutathione as a therapeutic agent or adjuvant therapy for a variety of diseases:

- **Supplementation:** While direct oral supplementation of glutathione has limits owing to low absorption, several researchers are investigating techniques to indirectly raise glutathione levels via precursor substances such as N-acetylcysteine (NAC) or alpha-lipoic acid.

- **Clinical treatments:** Clinical treatments targeted at restoring glutathione levels may be investigated as prospective therapy in specific conditions characterized by decreased glutathione levels, such as HIV/AIDS, chronic liver disorders, or cystic fibrosis.

Research And Studies

Scientific research is always looking at the relationship between glutathione levels and illness prevention or management:

- **Clinical studies:** Several clinical studies are being conducted to evaluate the usefulness of glutathione in alleviating symptoms or preventing the advancement of illnesses such as Parkinson's, Alzheimer's, cardiovascular disease, and cancer.

• **Cellular and Animal Studies:** Research in cellular and animal models often reveals glutathione's ability to reduce illness-related oxidative stress and halt disease development. These researches lay the ground for future human trials.

• **Molecular Mechanisms:** Understanding how glutathione works at the molecular level allows researchers to pinpoint its exact functions in various illnesses, enabling them to target particular pathways for treatments.

The role of glutathione in disease prevention and possible therapeutic uses is varied and expanding. Unlocking glutathione's full therapeutic potential may lead to novel techniques for preventing, managing, or even curing a variety of chronic illnesses as research advances.

CHAPTER 5

Factors Affecting Glutathione Levels

Certainly! Glutathione plays an important role in the body's defensive system. Here's a detailed look at the elements that influence its levels:

Genetics

• Genetic predispositions play an important role in defining an individual's baseline glutathione levels. Variations in genes encoding glutathione synthesis and recycling enzymes, such as glutathione peroxidases and glutathione transferases, might influence glutathione production and use.

• Certain genetic variations or polymorphisms may limit the body's capacity to efficiently produce or recycle glutathione. For example, mutations in the genes responsible for creating glutathione-metabolizing enzymes, such as GSTM1 or GSTP1, may impair an individual's capacity to maintain appropriate glutathione levels.

Lifestyle Choices

• **Diet:** A well-balanced diet rich in nutrients such as sulfur-containing amino acids (cysteine, methionine), vitamins (especially vitamins C and E), and minerals (selenium, zinc) is essential for promoting glutathione production. Garlic, onions, cruciferous vegetables, and some fruits help to increase glutathione levels.

• **Exercise:** Regular physical activity may boost glutathione levels. Excessive or intense exercise may temporarily diminish glutathione levels owing to oxidative stress, but moderate exercise may enhance glutathione synthesis. Consistent moderate exercise, on the other hand, boosts total antioxidant defenses.

• **Stress Management:** By increasing oxidative stress, chronic stress may decrease glutathione levels. Stress-reduction practices such as mindfulness, meditation, and proper sleep may aid in maintaining healthy glutathione levels.

Environmental Influences

• **Toxins and pollutants:** Exposure to environmental toxins, pollutants, heavy metals (such as lead, mercury, and arsenic) and chemicals (such as pesticides and air pollutants) may decrease glutathione levels since the body utilizes it to neutralize and remove these hazardous compounds.

• **Lifestyle habits:** Smoking, excessive alcohol intake, and secondhand smoke exposure may all lower glutathione levels owing to increased oxidative stress and the body's increased requirement for antioxidants to battle the detrimental effects of these activities.

Understanding these aspects is crucial for those who want to boost their glutathione levels. Lifestyle adjustments such as eating a balanced diet, controlling stress, and avoiding pollutants may all have a good influence on glutathione production and contribute to general health and well-being.

CHAPTER 6

Glutathione Supplementation

Glutathione, an important antioxidant, may be supplemented, perhaps providing health advantages. Understanding the forms, dosage, administration, and other variables is critical for optimal usage.

Forms Of Supplementation

1. Glutathione is available in a variety of forms, including capsules, pills, and liquid preparations. However, the effectiveness of oral supplementation is disputed owing to absorption issues. When taken orally, glutathione may be broken down in the digestive system before reaching circulation, decreasing its bioavailability.

2. **Glutathione Liposomal:** Liposomal formulations encapsulate glutathione inside lipid molecules to improve absorption. These may boost bioavailability

over standard oral supplements by protecting the chemical throughout the digestive process.

3. Intravenous or intramuscular administration: Glutathione injection bypasses the digestive system, resulting in increased absorption rates. Glutathione is often administered intravenously or intramuscularly by medical practitioners to treat certain health disorders or to quickly enhance its levels in the body.

Dosage And Administration

Glutathione dosage is complicated and varies depending on individual requirements, health circumstances, and supplementation methods.

1. Dosages for oral supplementation generally vary from 250 to 1,000 mg per day. However, because of issues regarding absorption, greater dosages may be required to obtain the intended benefits.

2. **Injections:** In general, intravenous or intramuscular delivery is done under medical supervision. Healthcare experts recommend dosage and frequency, which vary depending on the ailment being treated.

Considerations And Risks

1. Bioavailability is one of the most difficult aspects of using oral glutathione supplements. Digestive enzymes, stomach acid, and the structure of the chemical may all reduce its efficiency.

2. Glutathione supplements are usually thought to be safe for most individuals when used in adequate dosages. However, some people may develop minor side effects such as stomach pain, bloating, or allergic responses.

3. **Drugs:** Glutathione supplements may interfere with or reduce the effectiveness of certain drugs. Before beginning supplementation, it is critical to

check with a healthcare practitioner, particularly if you are taking drugs for certain health issues.

4. Long-term Use: The long-term consequences of glutathione supplementation are currently being studied. Further research on long-term high-dose use and associated side effects is needed.

5. Individual Differences: Individual responses to glutathione supplementation might vary depending on hereditary variables, health state, and lifestyle choices.

Before beginning glutathione supplementation, it is critical to understand these subtleties. It is best to get specialized advice from a healthcare expert to identify the best form, dose, and any hazards associated with supplements.

CHAPTER 7

Foods That Boost Glutathione

Glutathione, an important antioxidant, may be raised by food. Although eating glutathione-rich meals may not directly increase its levels in the body owing to digestion and absorption issues, some nutrients help in its creation. Concentrating on these nutrients aids the body's natural glutathione production.

Natural Sources In The Diet

A variety of foods provide ingredients that aid in glutathione formation. Sulfur-rich foods like garlic, onions, and cruciferous vegetables like broccoli, Brussels sprouts, and kale are examples. These foods include sulfur-containing chemicals such as cysteine and methionine, both of which are required for glutathione formation.

Glutathione levels are also increased by meals rich in selenium, such as Brazil nuts, sunflower seeds, and seafood. Selenium is an essential cofactor for glutathione peroxidase, an enzyme that interacts with glutathione in antioxidant defense.

Fruits like avocados, oranges, and strawberries, as well as vegetables like spinach and asparagus, include vitamins C and E, which both help the body's glutathione function.

Dietary Habits For Increased Levels

Including a variety of these items in one's diet helps promote the body's natural glutathione synthesis. A well-balanced diet rich in vegetables, fruits, nuts, seeds, and lean proteins provides a wide range of nutrients that aid in glutathione production.

Choosing whole, minimally processed meals gives a larger intake of critical elements for glutathione formation.

Cooking techniques may also have an influence on nutrient retention; softly steaming or sautéing veggies helps retain their nutritious content.

Recipes And Meal Ideas

Combining these glutathione-boosting foods may result in healthful and delectable meals. A salad with leafy greens, avocado, sunflower seeds, and citrus fruits, for example, has a variety of nutrients that promote glutathione formation.

A stir-fry with broccoli, garlic, onions, and lean protein sources like chicken or tofu is another choice. This not only has a variety of tastes, but it also includes nutrients that help with glutathione production.

Smoothies made with spinach, kale, berries, and a sprinkling of nuts or seeds may be a nutrient-dense snack that helps boost glutathione levels.

Individuals might increase their body's natural glutathione levels by adopting dietary habits that prioritize certain items and combining them into diverse meals. This promotes general health and antioxidant capacity.

While nutrition is important, other variables such as lifestyle, environmental exposures, and genetic predispositions also have an impact on glutathione levels in the body.

CHAPTER 8

Glutathione And Skin Health

Glutathione, dubbed the "master antioxidant," is critical to sustaining overall health and well-being. Its effect and possible advantages have gotten a lot of attention in the world of skincare. Let us now look at Chapter 8: Glutathione and Skin Health.

Antioxidant Effects On The Skin

The antioxidant capabilities of glutathione are critical for skin health. It scavenges free radicals caused by UV radiation, pollution, stress, and other environmental variables as an antioxidant. Glutathione protects skin cells from oxidative damage by neutralizing free radicals, possibly reducing the aging process. This technique also aids in the maintenance of skin elasticity and suppleness, which contributes to a young look.

Skin Whitening And Anti-Aging Claims

One of the more contentious features of glutathione in skincare is its alleged skin whitening and anti-aging properties. Some anecdotal evidence and limited research show that glutathione may help lighten skin by preventing the formation of melanin, the pigment responsible for skin color. This is said to minimize hyperpigmentation, resulting in a brighter complexion. A more thorough study, however, is required to definitively support these assertions.

In terms of anti-aging properties, glutathione's capacity to combat oxidative stress is critical. The breakdown of collagen and elastin in the skin caused by oxidative stress contributes to wrinkles and sagging. As an antioxidant, glutathione aids in the fight against stress, potentially slowing the aging process by preserving the structural proteins of the skin.

Topical Application

While glutathione pills or intravenous injections are routinely utilized for their systemic benefits, the usage of glutathione in topical skincare products has gained popularity. Some skincare formulations use glutathione as a main component in creams, serums, and lotions, claiming to provide immediate skin benefits. However, the effectiveness of topical glutathione remains a point of contention among specialists owing to issues with absorption and skin stability.

Further study on the effectiveness, appropriate dose, and long-term benefits of topical glutathione is necessary. Factors such as formulation, concentration, and delivery systems all have a substantial influence on its capacity to permeate the skin and provide the claimed benefits.

Understanding the subtleties of glutathione's involvement in skincare is a constantly expanding field of study. While its antioxidant qualities are promising, more extensive research is needed to confirm and fully comprehend its potential in improving skin health and treating particular dermatological issues.

CHAPTER 9

Controversies And Myths Surrounding Glutathione

Debunking Common Myths

1. **Oral Absorption:** There is a common misconception that oral glutathione supplements are poorly absorbed. While raw glutathione may not be well absorbed, some precursors or boosters such as N-acetylcysteine (NAC) or alpha-lipoic acid might indirectly raise glutathione levels.

2. **Skin Lightening:** The effects of glutathione on skin lightening are debatable. Some believe it may brighten skin tone, however, the scientific data is equivocal. Its antioxidant qualities and suppression of melanin formation may have skin-lightening benefits, but additional study is required.

3. Some people claim glutathione produces quick benefits. However, because of different body

composition, metabolism, and general health, its effects might vary from person to person. Consistent usage over time may be required to see substantial results.

Misconceptions About Supplementation

1. **High Doses Are Always Better:** Excessive glutathione consumption may not always be good. Excessive doses may disturb the body's natural equilibrium and perhaps create negative effects, therefore it's critical to keep to approved levels.

2. **One-Size-Fits-All Approach:** Not everyone requires or reacts to glutathione supplementation in the same manner. Its efficacy may be influenced by factors such as heredity, health circumstances, and lifestyle. A healthcare practitioner can help you establish the right dose and if you need to supplement.

Risks And Side Effects

1. Unanticipated effects: Despite being a natural chemical, glutathione supplementation may cause undesirable effects in certain people. Allergic reactions, stomach pain, and even aggravation of some illnesses are possible side effects.

2. Pharmaceuticals: Glutathione supplements may interfere with pharmaceuticals such as chemotherapy treatments or nitroglycerin. Before beginning supplementation, it is critical to contact a healthcare practitioner, particularly if you are receiving treatment or using drugs daily.

3. Long-Term consequences: The long-term consequences of glutathione supplementation have not been well investigated. As a result, depending on supplements excessively without sufficient counsel and knowledge of possible hazards may result in unanticipated health difficulties.

Addressing these issues and myths allows people to make more educated choices regarding glutathione supplementation and fosters a better awareness of its true advantages and limits. It is always best to consult with a healthcare expert before beginning any supplement regimen.

CHAPTER 10

Future Directions And Research

Because of its importance in a variety of physiological processes, glutathione is still the topic of substantial investigation. Ongoing research aims to improve our knowledge of its mechanics and prospective uses in a variety of fields:

Ongoing Studies

Numerous active researches are investigating various elements of glutathione. Beyond traditional knowledge, research is looking at its effects on mental health, neurological illnesses, cancer prevention, and metabolic diseases. Scientists are looking into its effect on gene expression, cell signaling, and even its potential as an adjuvant in cancer treatment or a therapeutic agent in neurological illnesses like Parkinson's and Alzheimer's.

Emerging Trends In Glutathione Research

One new theme in glutathione research is the investigation of innovative delivery mechanisms to improve glutathione absorption and bioavailability. To enhance its transport into cells and tissues, researchers are researching nanotechnology-based delivery methods, liposomal encapsulation, and other novel ways. Furthermore, research is being conducted to better understand the interaction between glutathione and the gut microbiota, as well as how gut health affects glutathione levels and vice versa.

Potential Discoveries

Researchers anticipate discovering additional activities and regulatory mechanisms connected with glutathione as technology and scientific approaches progress. This might entail discovering particular genetic markers that regulate glutathione production or investigating the possibilities of customized therapy in which glutathione levels could play an important role.

Furthermore, given the increased interest in antioxidants and anti-aging drugs, the identification of more powerful and effective glutathione analogs or derivatives might pave the way for the creation of improved therapeutic approaches.

The knowledge of glutathione's complex functions in health and illness is predicted to grow as research advances, possibly opening up new possibilities for therapeutic therapies and preventative healthcare.

This investigation into the future of glutathione research highlights the enormous potential for discoveries and uses that might alter health, wellness, and a variety of scientific areas. Further research and novel methodologies are anticipated to provide new insights into glutathione's multifunctional capabilities and their implications for human health and disease management.

Conclusion

Certainly! Glutathione is an important antioxidant found in almost every cell in the human body. It is essential in many physiological functions, and its levels are an indicator of general health and well-being. We've looked at the many different aspects of glutathione throughout this tutorial.

Glutathione, a tripeptide made up of three amino acids—cysteine, glutamic acid, and glycine—acts as a powerful antioxidant, protecting cells from oxidative stress and damage. Its main functions include detoxification, immunological support, and cellular protection. Endogenous glutathione synthesis occurs in the body, with genetics, lifestyle, and environmental variables all impacting its production.

Glutathione is undeniably important in sustaining health and vigor. Its importance is shown by its participation in several biological processes.

Despite its critical importance, disputes and misunderstandings about its supplementation exist. Understanding the facts, dispelling misconceptions, and appreciating the possible advantages and drawbacks of glutathione supplementation are all critical stages toward fully realizing its potential.

Glutathione's importance extends well beyond its antioxidant activity; it is essential in disease prevention, immunological support, and skin health. While continuing study continues to uncover its many roles, its importance cannot be understated.

As research uncovers the complexity of glutathione production, metabolism, and its impact on numerous areas of health, it is critical to approach supplementation and application with caution, taking individual requirements and health circumstances into account.

Finally, the breadth of glutathione's influence on human health emphasizes its significance.

Recognizing its functions, investigating its potential in illness prevention, and grasping the elements that control its levels may all help to improve health and well-being.

Understanding glutathione is not just a scientific endeavor, but it is also a critical component in harnessing its potential for improving health outcomes and general well-being.

THE END

56